When you do not know the nature of the malady, leave it to nature; do not strive to hasten matters. For either nature will bring about the cure or it will itself reveal clearly what the malady really is.

- Avicenna

To my wife and daughters:

Ahya' Hasni
Naila Huda
Haneen Huda

Preamble

Today's world is complex. It is partly because human beings have become much more inter-connected. With the advent of technology, social media, satellites and smartphones, we experience the spread of news and updates from one corner of the world to the other within seconds. Globalisation phenomenon has also set the stage for competitive and "disruptive" changes in various industries.

This world without borders has also changed the approach to doctoring, and the degree of responsibility that patients have towards their own health. In this information-rich and data-driven age, many patients are better-informed and inclined to know more about the updates and advancement in the medical field. This is so that they can explore the myriad of options and benefits from various available treatments. Realising that, it is no longer the case where patients are rendered at the receiving end, doing what's being told by their medical professionals. It is, instead, about partnership in trying to optimise the health the patients hope to achieve.

For the junior doctors, such change is not necessarily easy to handle. With the constant juggle between training pathways, clinical work challenges and keeping the impetus to continue doctoring, the concept of shared health goals and therapeutic partnership with patients can be the least of the focus. This book is written to share with both, the junior doctors and the patients about the dynamics of two different worlds. Hopefully, by doing so, the therapeutic partnership between doctors and patients can be bolstered.

There are several questions that this book will try to address. These include:
1. How can doctors adjust the way they manage and treat patients?

2. The perspective that can be adopted by trainees and junior doctors, going through training pathways.
3. How to look after our own health?
4. How should we define the concept of well-being?
5. What has been the development in several important areas of health challenges?
6. What can be the unique way our society can contribute to other fellow human beings through the advancement of medical knowledge?

This book is designed to be a mix of science as well as thoughts and opinions. It is also designed to be a go-to book for inspiration, tranquillity, human experience as well as thought-provoking topics. It is certainly not a book that provides definitive solutions, instead, it serves as a foundation for readers to think more about the topics and formulate further thoughts in each specific area. The book also has several pictures of personally captured, beautiful scenery in New Zealand to give a rest to the mind and the soul of the readers.

Enjoy!

Contents:

- Secrets to Success.

- Being A Palpably Alive Doctor.

- A look at the Concept of Education – The Paradoxical Law of Deficiency to Generate Breakthroughs.

- Career and Life, Journey of Medical Training.

- Well-Being, The Centre of Living.

- How to Be Healthy.

- Advance Care Plan, Communication That Matters.

- Clinical Decision Making and Cognitive Biases.

- The Best of Contribution, Filling Life with an Everlasting sense of Giving.

- Updates in the Field of Cancer.

- Revisiting the World of Mental Health.

- Structure and Approach to Care for Patients – A Guide for Interns.

Secrets to Success.

"When I let go of what I am, I become what I might be."– Lao Tzu

People say, to be successful, we need to learn from those who have already achieved success and created success stories. While success in life is a dynamic goal, it also forms a culture. What defines success differs between each person - it can be from the smallest of achievements to a tremendous milestone that one achieves in life.

If we study people who made significant achievements in history - from world billionaires, professionals, social engineers, philanthropists and many more, there are unifying formulae that group them together. These formulae are so consistent and for that matter, they make success reproducible for people who embody them.

I wish to begin this book by outlining these formulae. They are from a review and my analysis of the behaviours and principles of successful people. It is hoped that they will also make anybody who is pursuing the career of medicine and wanting to be health professional becomes successful and lives beyond the pressure of healthcare demand.

What are the determinants of human growth and success?

If you study people like Bill Gates, Warren Buffet, Jim Rohn, Tony Robbins, Ray Dalio, Jack Ma and innumerable more people in the history, these people EMBODIED these formulae that I call "the culture and habit to success."

Let us have a look at the following list and try to imagine and embody them in our life.

1. Successful people NEVER give excuses, instead, they always find ways. They don't complain about

problems but they see every problem as an opportunity. If we convert every problem to opportunity, life will become amazing. Human creativity will grow exponentially. The change of focus from problem-oriented to opportunity-oriented pushes us to find the solution that will be a great offer to the society. It changes our state from being a pessimist and victim of a situation to a master of a new idea. It boosts our confidence and definitely our action.

2. They have an absolute belief. What is this absolute belief? It is what we call as faith. Faith is when we do, embody and live by what we believe even without yet seeing the eventual result. So much so, when hurdles come, obstacles appear, things seem impossible, the conviction of our inner voices tells us to keep going. As a saying in the Forrest Gump movie, *"I keep going."* Successful people don't ruminate about what happens to them, instead, they feel everything happens FOR them. They find meanings behind everything.

3. They are humble and they have a sense of gratitude. Research shows that gratitude for each and every component of life that we experience contributes to the feeling of happiness.

4. They are very charitable. Giving and gratitude will make you wealthy and this is definitely proven by many people.

5. They have rituals, standards and strategies. It is a culture shift from *"I can do"* to *"I must do"*, a transformation from *"I shall"* to *"I must."*

6. They make things happen NOW! If you read books like *Think and Grow Rich* by Napoleon Hill or *Unleash the Power Within* by Tony Robbins, you will realise that the biggest difference that makes someone successful and not is a difference in ACTION. Faster action means faster result, it opens to an earlier and bigger opportunity.

7. They make the investment for their personal growth and development as the utmost life investment.

8. They are risk-takers but they take the risks with the right psychology and strategies.

9. They make decisions and act on their decisions.

10. They create the new self-talk in their minds that negates all negativity and instead, they say, *"Why not you and why not now?"*.

11. They face and overcome their fears. They welcome rejection and keep on trying.

12. They have financial discipline - save and invest first, spend what's left.

13. They have mentors, they read books and they take actions.

14. They add values to this world and create LEGACIES.

15. Their focus is helping people and adding values to others' lives.

16. They went through hardships.

17. They DO what others DON'T.

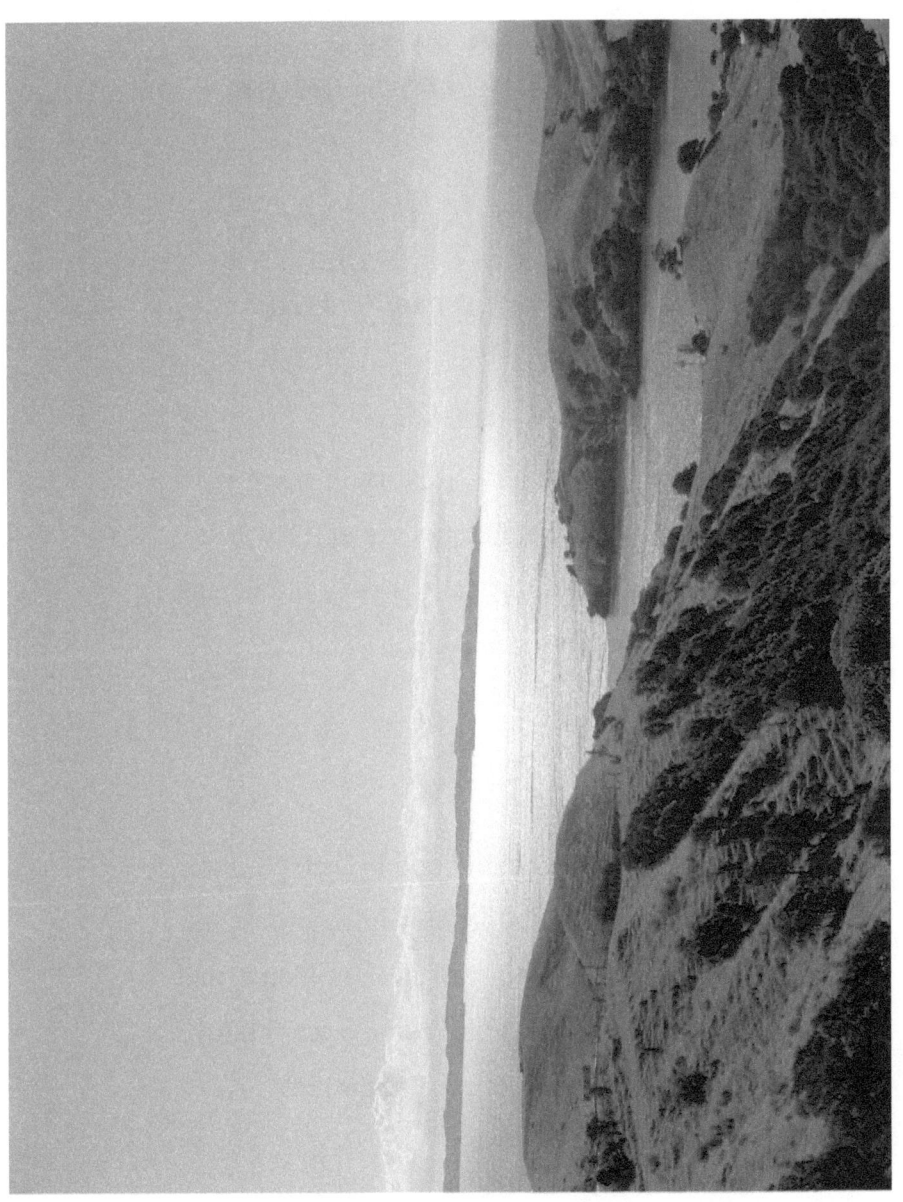

Coromandel, New Zealand

Being A Palpably Alive Doctor.

"The good physician treats the disease; the great physician treats the patient who has the disease."- William Osler

When I was a teen, medicine was never my cup of tea. It was not an area familiar to me and I was not from a family of doctors. Just seeing blood and needles was enough to make my stomach feel queasy.

In saying this, during my childhood to college years, humanity and human relationships have been close to my heart. Listening to people's problems and stories, leading, motivating and being a team player were part and parcels of what I went through.

The passing of my late uncle from gastric adenocarcinoma brought me closer to the reality of death and opened up a very personal experience to me. It was probably one of the first triggers that led me to choose this profession eventually.

When I was sixteen, my brother was caught in an accident at a training camp. He sustained an extra-capsular neck of femur fracture. Several cannulated screws were inserted and he was lucky that there was no sub-capital, intra-capsular fracture. If he sustained the latter, then he might need to live with a hip replacement at a very young age. While current data suggested long-term durability of hip replacement, there will be long-term risk of needing revision and also risk of endo-prosthesis infection.

Following the operation, I helped mum to care for him for several weeks until he was able to walk steadily again. I remembered though, when he was hospitalised, there was another patient next to his bed. He was caught in a severe truck accident and he was lucky to be alive. He sustained a significant degloving injury and a severely comminuted fracture of his left leg. What I could see was the external fixator on the outside, trying to maintain the length of the leg while awaiting further surgery for an intramedullary nail, open reduction and internal fixation(ORIF) and eventually skin grafting.

The experience of being in the hospital for several days to support my family pushed me a bit further to understand medicine and the life of doctors and nurses.

I went to the preparatory program, chose medicine most likely due to the trend and popularity during that time, how naive! During that time, I did not yet have the comprehensive idea of why did I want to do medicine? My standard answer in the interview was, *"I want to help and assist the people in need."* It's noble-sounding but not profound, it could be ignorant too!

Eventually, I got the offer to pursue my medical degree and flew to New Zealand. This was when my perspective started to change. New Zealand is a beautiful country and populated by supportive and friendly people. Studying health sciences here led me to love the subjects. I started to learn about body systems and I was amazed at how they function. Gradually, I started to have a better grasp of the biomedical sciences. Deep inside, I told myself that I should embody this profession as part of my life through which I could connect with my Creator.

What was amazing in Otago, from early on, we were introduced to patient-centred medicine. Communication skills and exploring the illnesses of patients via the Calgary-Cambridge Model were part of the backbones of the clinical skills. I didn't quite understand this rationale then. It was unfathomable how communication skills formed a huge part in passing the exam and becoming a doctor. I would have thought knowledge and procedural skills stood as the priority to developing competency in doctors.

Six years of medical school passed very quickly. While feeling truly inspired and with the strong passion to start doctoring, I could recall an advice from the Dean of Clinical School. In his advice, he mentioned about the three things that graduates would need to remember as we embarked on the journey as junior doctors. The first thing was to **recognise our fear**. There would be many instances where a clinical situation would bring us to face our own fear. The challenge would be to recognise and acknowledge it. From there, growth would happen and we would eventually master the art of dealing with this emotion.

The second thing was to **be cautious of institutional thinking and workplace polarisation**. This did not specifically apply to medicine but could be applicable in the clinical workplace. Each hospital and in each department, there were departmental cultures and protocols that have been there for many years or even for generations. What could happen is people who came to work in the department got conditioned to this work behaviour and a departmental way of doing things. Sometimes, this could be at the expense of creativity, innovativeness and efficiency. What might be worse, for junior doctors, protocoled treatment pathway while could be good for patients, could also led young interns to follow blindly without understanding the reasons.

Thirdly, **commitment**. Medicine was all about commitment. Hard work, taking ownership of the cases, accountability, decisiveness were all the characters that needed to be developed as medical practitioners. The road won't be easy but, eventually, it would be rewarding.

Six years have now passed since I started working as a junior doctor. There were several areas that I felt make a big difference between a good doctor and a bad doctor. Putting it another way, what pushes one to be a palpably alive doctor? A doctor who connects and can deliver the best possible patient-doctor therapeutic relationship?

Is it competency, kindness, thoroughness or what exactly? I did an audit about this several years ago. I sent a set of questionnaires to a group of doctors and the same questionnaires to a group of nurses. Both groups were asked to rate the skills that made someone a good doctor. Amazingly, doctors and nurses had very different opinions about what's considered the most important skill to have. The nurse rated communication skills as the first one while the doctors put competency!

There are several areas that make up or define a person. A lot of doctors are very good at biomedical sciences. They use biomedical sciences and treat their patients. If patients are approached only with biomedical knowledge, then they become the object of the experiments. This is actually reflected from the meaning of the original word for patient itself, which is the object of an action.

This model of medicine reduces a person to **scientific knowledge**, taking away other dimensions that makes one a human being.

There is another dimension that is important. This is the **human identity** that makes someone who he or she is. Human identity comes from the blend of upbringings, culture, education, skills, religion, family and society that people live with over a period of time. *While biomedical sciences try to explain the process and the science of human existence, human identity is the existential meaning that evolves from these sciences.*

Therefore, to be a palpably alive doctor is to be a doctor who can bridge between the biomedical sciences and specific personal identity and meaning. It is a two-tier level of care with a condition that in the situation where there is no cure for the biomedical process, accentuating the "therapy" at the level of human identity remains of utmost importance.

Being able to include the two components in healthcare is what we call the art of medicine and personalised care. The interactions between the two domains of care can be illustrated in this particular experience of mine;

I met with Mary (non-de-plume), a 40-year-old lady who presented with acute respiratory failure. Mary was a lovely lady who's married to her husband and has a 14-year-old daughter. She worked as an administrator in one of the hospitals.

She was first diagnosed with breast cancer in 2015 with genotype ER/PR negative and HER2 positive. Unfortunately, her cancer progressed to metastatic disease and continued to progress despite several lines of chemotherapy and Pertuzumab/Trastuzumab therapy. Her course of breast cancer was aggressive with the first diagnosis of metastatic disease from initial diagnosis of breast cancer, measured in less than 1 year.

When I saw Mary, her cancer had reached the stage where further chemotherapy would not be useful and would only cause more toxicity to her body, jeopardising her quality of life.

From the biomedical perspective, there was nothing much that we could offer Mary because her cancer was incurable, but this was not the end of the story.

As mentioned, she has her family and her life that made who she was. The question was, how do we support her in reconciling her colours of life with the current existential threat? It has to be with good communication, counselling and discussion about what makes her quality of life and what her wishes are.

Hence, we talked to her that the goal and direction of treatment changes from trying to cure her to helping her to be as comfortable as she could. We discussed with her about making a plan for herself and her family, how she wanted to be cared for until the end as well as how she could optimise the short, meaningful time with her loved ones.

She made a plan to buy a birthday gift in advance for her daughter so that her daughter can open it in a few months' time when she would no longer be around.....

Being able to feel where a patient is at in their journey of illness makes a doctor alive in the heart of the patient. This is what constitutes a good and humane doctoring skill.

The success of any prescribed treatment is dependent upon the adherence by patients. To achieve adherence, it partly relies on how good health professionals can relate to the **human identity and meaning**. When illness befalls somebody, the degree of impact relates to how damaging it can be to this element. The more jeopardised it is, the more people will go to try to find the cure. Knowing this, doctors who are skilful at using this aspect as a leverage can change patients' health behaviour.

The question is, what can the doctors do to relate better with human identity and meaning?

Biomedical sciences fall short in giving us this perspective. They do not answer the question such as *"Why me?"*. They do not engage with human emotions. They do not address meanings that people put in their lives.

Literature and real-life encounters are the two sources that can teach us about this connection. Literature is great because it conveys the real-life emotions of the *writers*. It tells the true stories, how they unravel and the journeys that different people take. It describes different people's lives, what's important to them, the interaction between them and their diseases and what eventually becomes their coping strategies. Real-life experience is the other source. Whether in a clinical setting or in our daily relationships, real-life experience enriches us with perspectives and help us to understand the human dynamics better.

Why are these sources important? If we take a look at the job of doctors, doctors from the time of internship and onwards go through rigorous training processes. The clinical duty can be very hectic leading to the time spent with each person being very short. The hours spent in the hospital are long, the time spent with family, friends and society is minimal. In a way, this creates a cocooned environment that is detached from the human daily life, stories and dynamics. What we get is only the small window of patient's life at a very limited time.

While some argue that to be competent doctors, the hours and for that matter, rigorous training is important, detachment from the normal life can make the ability to gel the biomedical sciences with the human identity quite precarious. This is clearly seen when doctors are not comfortable to discuss and address in detail patients' emotions, using jargon language and being less sensitive when talking about delicate issues with them. In a global society now, patients are made up of people with different cultures. Being less informed about different cultures and traditions make some doctors to be culturally incompetent and this can have negative ramifications on the health outcome of patients.

Therefore, learning through literature and networking outside the clinical arena, will keep health professionals at touch with humanity and help to bridge the two elements of care more successfully.

The paternalistic style in medical care is now well-outdated. Patients nowadays are more knowledgeable. At the same time, they run the risk of being misled by the unverified, abundance of information out-there. Patient-centred medicine was proposed in an effort to put more responsibility and appreciate the autonomy of patients in deciding care for themselves. While this sounds elegant, there is also an inherent problem. Being only patient-centred might mean honouring all of the patients' wishes at the expense of clinical and ethical aptness. Somebody may want every possible intervention despite its futility and it will be difficult to draw the clinically appropriate boundary. Should health professionals be pressured to attempt something despite impossible outcome? The art of doctoring and the patient-doctor relationship, for me, involve clinical stewardship and guidance. It is not exclusively patient-centred medicine, instead, settles in the arena of clinical guidance and negotiation. Our job as doctors is to provide guidance as to what will be the best approach, investigations, treatments and also to facilitate patients to reach to sound decisions. When it comes to the ceiling of care, patients are to be informed about what is appropriate and what is not. At the same time, health professionals need to be protected from performing resuscitation or approving treatment when deemed to be causing more harm.

Clinical guidance is what is often found missing in our care for patients. In the medical world, we have this term WICOS - who is the chief of the ship? When a person is very sick, attention is drawn from a lot of specialities. While this can be good, it can also be dangerously counterproductive. The reason is, everybody looks and only looks at the specific body system related to their speciality. Nobody combines all these together and look at the person as a whole. This can be a recipe for total disaster!

Moreover, losing WICOS can mean a loss in connecting at the level of human identity and meaning. Have you ever wondered, when your kidney is not working, your heart is playing up, your bowels go into ileus due to ascites, what springs to mind is not how each of these organs is doing in separation? It is, what do all these mean and how will these impact on my existence and my family, job, relationship, friends, quality and activities of daily life?

Hopefully, by polishing the two elements of clinical care, we can all be a more competent, caring and a palpably alive doctor in the heart of our patients.

Elements of A Good Care:

Biomedical Sciences.

Connection with Human Identity and Meaning.

A Look at the Concept of Education - The Paradoxical Law of Deficiency to Generate Breakthroughs.

"The difference between a successful person and others is not lack of strength nor a lack of knowledge but rather a lack of will."– Vince Lombardi

I met with a couple of patients, whom accentuated my belief on certain philosophy of education and what makes a person able to add values to the world we are living in.

The first one, is Mr Smith (non-de plume). Mr Smith was a 70-year-old man, who lived in Papua New Guinea. He owned a television station over-there. He never received a formal education and spent most of his time sailing between Papua New Guinea and New Zealand. He used to have a modified boat as his place of living. I found this man unique, despite no formal education, he managed to open a television station to serve the people in Papua New Guinea.

Few days after meeting him, I met with another patient, Mr Brown. He was a 60-year-old man with a background of Spinal Muscular Atrophy and suffered from tetraplegia. The only movement he has was from the neck upwards and his right index finger. This man's life relied upon two full-time carers to assist with his daily life. You know what, he owned and managed his software company with his right index finger. Amazing!

Yes, there are many educated people that contribute and add values to the world, but, often those who made life-changing games and revolutionary contribution were not those born out of the formal education system.

People like Richard Branson, Tony Robbins, Steve Jobs, Bill Gates were not graduates at their young age. They were not the product of linear education system i.e. going through schools and eventually received the scrolls.

This proves a huge and vital point. There is a mismatch between the current education system and the exploration of human innate potentials. The education system has been designed to be an industrial education system, with machinery conception. It has been designed to channel the human resources to different industrial needs.

I agree with Sir Ken Robinson, an elite in creative schooling and education. Human beings are organic, their developments are organic. What's needed in their education is not conformity, one size fits all, rather, we need diversity and personalisation of the education. Each and every kid that grows up has their hidden talents, enormous potentials. What's needed is creating a condition that allows for the potentials to develop. Education should be a process of exploring and learning rather than dominated by the examinations.

It's not then surprising that some people that dropped out from school or universities flourish and succeed tremendously. They broke-out from an industrial education system that conformed people to specific fields and suppressing them of their in-born potentials.

It interests me too, to learn the pattern of how human deficiency, can in fact be the strength that pushes us all to make a breakthrough success and progress. Think about it again, a lot of the time, people make big achievements when they are scarce in resources. Unstable family background, poverty, illness, etc were the kind of colours we would see in the background. Out of these deficiencies, these people gained strengths and created legacies.

Amazing, it is the deficiencies rather than necessarily more resources that determine success! Indeed, a breakthrough comes from a deficient state but with ourselves being resourceful.

Career and Life, Journey of Medical Training.

"Do not go where the path may lead, go instead where there is no path and leave a trail."–
Ralph Waldo Emerson

Medical profession is one of the many noble professions. It goes without saying that the field and the profession are fundamental to human health, longevity and the asset to sustainable human civilisation.

Due to that reason, one of the indicators for a developed nation is a good and sustainable healthcare system.

There are a lot of reasons for why people choose to do medicine or health-related professions. In many of these reasons, if you ask from the nurses right to the consultants, the noble reason to alleviate suffering and to help people will always be there, directly or indirectly. What this tells us is, humanity is in fact at the heart and should always be made to be the heart of medical practice.

While the purpose is there, this fire of hope tends to fade, disappear or got stolen going through the medical career and following the stereotypical stream of training. The hours of working, the hostile senior-junior doctors relationship in some places, the medicolegal pressure from patients or their families, late presentations leading to very sick patients, unprofessional behaviours of some doctors at all levels, absence of mentoring or clinical leadership can be the factors that lay to rest this purpose.

Eventually, the character and personality of these high-spirited doctors falter. They become institutionalised in their way of thinking. They can become insolent to their colleagues and their juniors, impolite to their patients. The humanity that should be the driving force to care being provided is not felt by anyone around. The nature of the job has changed the doctors completely and made them drown in this system. Of course, this does not apply to all doctors or nurses, some turn out to be fine due to their resilience.

There is also another dimension to this. As a physician trainee in NZ, I attended the annual Trainees' Day. In 2016, one of the topics that were discussed was training pathway. When we join any particular training, there is a pathway. For the physicians in Australia and NZ, it is a 36-months of basic training, followed by the RACP physician exam, and then, another 3 to 4 years of advanced training. What interested me though, as the presenter who was also the RACP Chairman for NZ explained this, he highlighted the fact that there are life events that go along as we train. There can be a cost to our training. It can be less time spent with our children growing up, broken marriages and divorces. It can also be a life-ending illness.

Talking about the latter, it reminded me of the book I recently read entitled *When Breath Becomes Air* by Paul Kalanithi. Paul is a young neurosurgeon-neuroscientist who was a few months away from becoming a Professor of Neurosurgery. The training to become one in the United States, as you can imagine, involves a rigorous training and hours of working. Going to work early morning and coming back late at night has been the bread and butter for him for years. His wife, Lucy was an internal medicine specialist. You could imagine how hectic life would be for them. Unfortunately, Paul was diagnosed with pulmonary adenocarcinoma. The battle against cancer with molecular targeted therapy and several lines of chemotherapy managed to prolong his survival by 12-18 months. Nevertheless, the brutality of the cancer did not allow for his life to go beyond that. It was well written and depicted the life aspect of doctors.

What this suggests, while doctoring is great, it is great because it touches the human heart. The training is challenging and hence, what is crucial is, for us to take care of ourselves, our family, our relationship and people around us. Certainly, resilience in training is important, but if it robs you and me of the sense of humanity, then we should ask ourselves again the purpose of our job in the first place.

Taking the Time-Off.

In medicine, there is a terminology called pulses paradoxus. In traditional cardiology or other medical textbooks, it is described as the accentuation in a decrement in systolic blood pressure in the situation where patients have cardiac tamponade, severe asthma with gas trapping, restrictive cardiomyopathy although less so in the chronic state. In oncology patients with metastasis to the pericardium and fluid accumulation, pulses paradoxus is what we partly look for clinically to determine cardiac tamponade.

It is in fact accentuation rather than a paradox because the blood pressure goes further than usual 8-10 mm Hg physiological drop during deep inspiration. In normal physiological state though, in Christchurch, we have proven that what in fact happens is the blood pressure goes up with deep inspiration, hence, this is a challenge to the theory in the medical textbooks.

Anyway, the concept of accentuation and paradox are very similar to our medical job. Persistence in doing our job without taking the time-off, contrary to the common belief, makes doctors' performance worse. The clinical decision-making becomes less critical, mistakes occur more frequently, the spirit to perform the job deteriorates. We put ourselves to be not just physically but also mentally fatigued.

I would argue that taking the time-off, paradoxically, will help you to become a better clinician. This is because, while you are off-work and engage with other parts of life, you learn medicine from a humanity angle, you keep your family energised and in shape, you bolster your connection with your community. These help to develop your maturity when treating your patients.

Collegiality.

Collegiality is important in medical practice. This is something that no medical textbooks will teach but in fact, what helps clinicians to survive in medical practice. Having colleagues that care and share the workloads, avoiding the blame game and empowering each other transform the delivery of care to a safer, accurate, effective and with less error.

Collegiality does not only apply at the same level. It should transcend vertically from junior practitioners to consultants, clinical directors and hospital leadership groups. It can be contradictory that while the nature of our job should mean that we provide tenderness, love and care for our patients, the culture of ABCD - assess, blame, critic and destroy is rampantly practiced in some clinical workplace.

Creating the environment that supports collegiality would certainly be the way forward. This is achieved in different ways in different places. In New Zealand for instance, we love the coffee break - it provides the opportunity for improved collegiality and care for each other. It is also a great opportunity to discuss clinical cases further and provides the opportunity for medical students to get better insights into what they envision their profession would be in the near future.

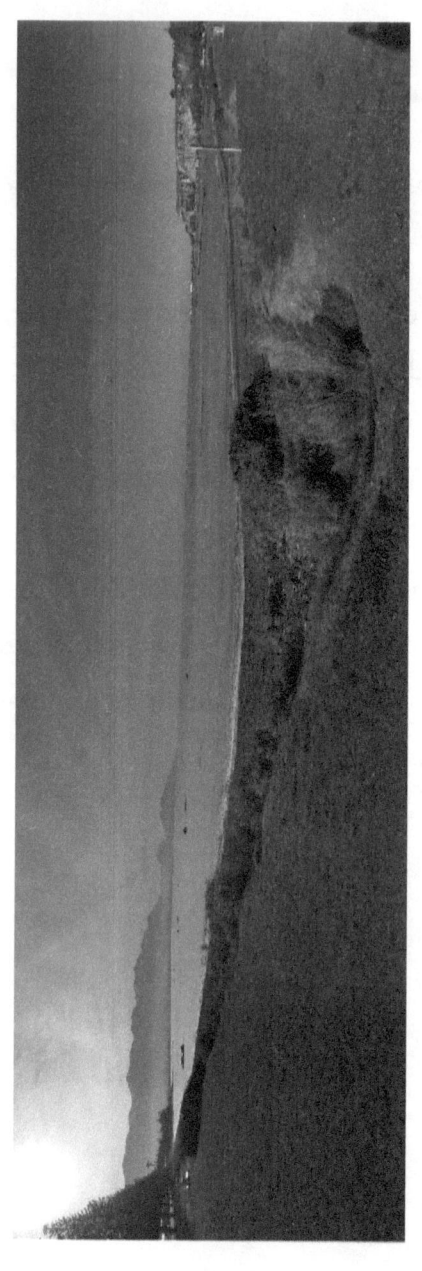

Lake Tekapo, NZ

Well-Being, The Centre of Living.

"Do not let what you cannot do interfere with what you can do."– John Wooden

All of us want a beautiful life. A beautiful life is a life where our dreams come through, our mind, our body, our spirit and our psychology resonate with each other. It gives us a sense of peace and empowerment inside. A beautiful life is not a life without challenges, rather, it is life with challenges that are dealt with positively and confidently. A beautiful and fulfilled life is a life where connections are made with families, friends, community and the society.

Undeniably, a beautiful and fulfilling life requires health. Health allows us to live long, to maintain a relationship, to achieve our dreams and to avoid sufferings as a result of physical or mental illnesses. Due to this, health becomes one of the most important elements in human life. It gives us some assurance to our existence. While health is one of the greatest wealth in this world, not everybody is born healthy. Those who are born healthy don't always stay healthy. Our health can deteriorate as each day goes by due to the complex interactions between our environment, social, upbringings and our genes.

While each day, we in the medical world advocate for preservation and maintenance of health, the reality is, people's health will deteriorate at some point.

Hence, could that mean our "Quality Life" is jeopardised because our health deteriorates? There is some truth in this. In medicine, medical doctors talk about optimisation of quality of life in the situation where patients are not at their best of health. When we cannot treat the diseases or illnesses, our focus shifts to the quality of life rather than the quantity of life. In health economics, we call this Quality-Adjusted Life-Years(QALY) gains.

But, what is meant by the optimisation of Quality of Life(QoL)? Should we think about optimisation of Quality of Life only when people are riddled with ailments? What are the actual determinants of good Quality of Life?

Quality of Life (QoL) is indeed very subjective and at the same time very personal from one person to the other. What's considered Quality of Life for a person could be the complete opposite to the other person. What this suggests is, the determinants of the QoL for each individual depends upon the possessions or achievements of what they considered important to their life. For instance, for one person, working fewer hours, having several cars and having good neighbours would be QoL. For the other person, having many kids and helping people around, would be counted as QoL.

This brings us to the notion of well-being. People achieve a quality life when they are in the state of well-being. What is well-being? This is, admittedly, a difficult question to answer. Many researchers now and in the past as well as philosophers including Aristotle attempted to define well-being but a lot of them ended up describing the aspects of well-being. So, we have social well-being, mental well-being, physical well-being, etc.

My personal view is, it is hard to define well-being because it is a type of feeling and a type of state that we are in. It is a feeling that comes from reconciliation of our heart, our mind and our body to the why, how and what in our life. It is about feeling well in ourselves in various aspects and feeling fulfilled. It is the connection of various aspects of our life that render us the sense of peace deep inside. Understanding this, well-being is, therefore, the pinnacle to living a quality life.

Why is this important? It is because, people can have diseases and illnesses but they can still maintain their state of well-being. People can be afflicted with torments of war but we can still help them to connect with their state of well-being.

It is an unfair call to say that people who are not completely healthy may not attain well-being. It is a right for each individual in whatever situation they are in, to be able to achieve this state. People in Syria, Palestine, Iraq and many other countries, might live in poor health status due to the wars that tore the countries apart. If we can help them to embody the feeling of well-being, then we would be able to link them to the state that even some rich countries and rich people might not acquire.

In the medical world nowadays, we provide a lot of care and treatments. As a result, people live longer, albeit with chronic medical conditions. We would see a 90-year-old with a mix of heart disease, kidney disease, diabetes, osteoporosis and other co-morbidities. A cocktail of medications keeps them alive although with feeble body and organ functions. In other words, they are frail. Some people at this age say, *"I had enough of the good life and there is nothing more I wish from this world."* What happens though, in the hospital, we still treat them knowing their wishes due to our medical obligations and ethics. Some people fall into depression, loneliness and the feeling of guilt from the need to be dependent on others.

Of course, some wish to continue for as long as they can since they still have their wish-list that is not yet fulfilled.

The medical world works on two notions, life-preserving treatment and optimisation of the Quality of Life. When pursuing life-preserving treatment, what sometimes can happen is, intensive medical treatment and medicalising the death and dying process. Despite the futility, we give it a go, just because we might be able to reverse the pathophysiology, albeit transiently.

I remember reading the book, *The Lost Art of Healing* by Bernard Lown. In one of the chapters, he explained how doctors before the invention of the stethoscope, put their ears onto the chest of the patients to listen to the heart and to the lung sounds. With the invention of technology, this human empathetic touch was lost. We use handheld echocardiogram to get more accurate bedside information of the function of the heart. This is all good provided that the art of humanity is also optimised and preserved. If teachers are the life-line of education, then the art of doctoring and caring for patients is the life-line of medicine.

So, with an ageing population, increase in life expectancy and medical intuition to treat and cure patients, is there anything new that we can add to bring about more values to our patients?

I think the answer is, yes. Since the reason for treatment and care provision has to do with humanity and caring for our fellow human beings, we can certainly do beyond our medications and multi-disciplinary support. I would suggest connecting our patients with and promoting the attainment of the state of well-being. Such is almost absent in many medical consultations. When we treat patients, we often either focus on the biomedical model treating diseases or the psycho-social model by providing multidisciplinary inputs.

What if we can include in our consultations, *"How's life for you at the moment?"*. What about *"Do you have the specific things in your life that would make you happy, lively, fulfilled and feel life is beautiful?"*. How about *"Are you in pursuit of reaching your dreams and at what stage are you in that?"*. What about asking *"Have you got a plan to convert your life to the fullest?"* or *"How is your social relationship, family relationship, work and performance?"*.

We often ask patients to have a bucket-list of things they wish to do when they are given bad news or diagnoses. What if we can generate this discussion regardless of health conditions? What if we can push them towards the state of well-being? What if we can suggest that they do not wait and instead, convert their lives immediately to attain the state of well-being?

After all, life and health are not only measured by length but more importantly, the quality that we have with the life that we are living. We have seen people asking to end their lives due to the sufferings even when they could still live for a long time. It is not saying this is right but extracting a reality that, what is most important to any human being is the state of well-being and living a quality life. For that matter, the wars and the injustices that can challenge the right for people's well-being, dignity and quality of life should be an international concern.

For instance, when we discuss heart-lung resuscitation, some patients would say "yes, regardless of the success and harm, I wish to be resuscitated." When we asked them carefully again about what they actually wanted, we would find that they wished for survival and preservation of the same body state prior to resuscitation. Nobody wants resuscitation, they want resuscitation because they believe resuscitation will bring them back to their healthy or previous state.

In summary, I believe if well-being is made a part of the discussion in medical consultations, we would be able to add huge values to our patients' lives. On top of treating our patients, we push them to find their state of well-being as we know in any spectrum of health, well-being is a right and a potential that everybody has and capable of achieving.

As a slogan I wish to coin, Well-Being is The Centre of Living...

How to Be Healthy - Medical Perspective.

"The knowledge of anything, since all things have causes, is not acquired or complete unless it is known by its causes." - Avicenna

The biggest industry in the world is undoubtedly health industry. Health is the key asset if we are speaking of financial or wealth terms. Everybody wants to not only be healthy but maintain the state of health. Due to that, there are many products, books, treatments and recommendations made by many, even sometimes by only God knows who and from where.

It is therefore not surprising for some products to be sold with a claim that everything could be cured by just taking them. Myth as it sounds, such claim only tries to reap monetary advantage out of the human hope to live as long and as healthy as possible.

Now, let us come to the facts and reality about health. Human health has three phases, ascending phase, plateau phase and descending phase. Ascending phase is the phase where we grow and build our body's physiological reserve. This process goes on until a certain age when it starts to plateau. After the period of plateau, degeneration starts to occur. Of course, congenital illnesses or familial illnesses are precluded from these typical stages.

What then influences health knowing the three phases? Certainly, health determinants are the variables that implicate directly or indirectly the phases we mentioned above whether at individual or population level.

So, what are these variables?

To understand these variables, we must first understand why we contract diseases. The medical textbooks, journals, reviews, observational and interventional studies suggest to us that diseases experienced by people are a result of interactions between several domains including human factor (genetics), the environment, occupational exposure, lifestyle, exercise and level of activities, health behaviours and upbringings. Socio-economic level and health literacy also play a part. The magnitude of interactions could be variable but essentially these are the determinants of diseases and health. Some of these are non-modifiable while others are modifiable.

Why is understanding these health determinants important? It is because attainment and maintenance of health involve alterations of the modifiable factors mentioned. Therefore, the reliable guides to health that you can follow are the guides that examine these factors. This is exactly what's been addressed in the field of preventive medicine.

So, how to be healthy?

1. **Exercise and Being Active** is one of the best ways to maintain your health. There is no doubt about this. It applies to kids right to frail elderlies. It applies from physical exercise to mental activeness.

2. **Eating moderately and eating good, nutritious food**. You will find in the market all sorts of diets - from Atkins' Diet to Paleo Diet. What we know, Mediterranean and Japanese diets are good and reduce the cardiovascular risk. Reduce simple sugar, limit table salt intake, reduce trans-fatty acid-containing food.

3. **Change the health behaviour**. Smoking cessation and reduction in alcohol intake for

those taking heavy amount of alcohol. Develop a good combination of nutritious food and exercise. Change the sedentary lifestyle.

4. **Nurture your family to create positive upbringings for your children.** This is important for the psychological well-being of our children. On top of literature evidence that suggests this, I personally noticed the same thing as I conducted a motivational talk to the youths of then aged 11 to 15 years old. In the Power of Imagination slot, I asked them, where would they see themselves in 10 years' time? Interestingly, most of the youths pointed to the ambitions that they could relate with in their families and these were mostly the occupation of their parents.

5. **Upgrade the socio-economic status partly through improvement in financial wellbeing**. Financial freedom and financial wellbeing can elevate families to a better socio-economic standard. This is important because they lead to more family time, better options for food, better education, and better lifestyle which would all affect our health. As Dalai Lama pointed out, *"Human beings are interesting, they work hard to become wealthy at the expense of their health, when they are wealthy they start then paying for their health."* Financial education is therefore paramount to avoid this and to allow for a better financial state.

6. **Engage with health agencies and services** and take the ownership of your own health. Health is about developing a partnership between yourself and your doctor. For that

reason, many countries have family medicine / general practitioners services so that the community members can receive longitudinal follow-up.

7. **Joining health screening program** for breast cancer, cervical cancer and colon cancer. Get an annual check-up for vascular risk factors such as diabetes, high cholesterol and blood pressure. As we know, the way to deal with cancer is early detection, prevention and early treatment whereas the best way to reduce the risk for heart attack, stroke, kidney dysfunction and fatty liver disease is by regulating all the risk factors early on.

8. **Increase your health literacy**. Given that health is the priceless entity in life, it has also developed into a very lucrative industry for

businesses. This has gone to the extent that products are being sold without evidence-based data to support their use. Some of the products could be detrimental to the kidneys and the liver. Things that people need to know is, their body physiology has its reserve. The supplements are usually not needed if they can get the nutrients from food. There is no need to get additional supplements if you are not malnourished. The key is to get the advice from your clinicians. The other thing that people need to be aware of is products with testimonial evidence. The preciousness of health means people should NEVER succumb their state of body function to not well-researched products.

So, those are the pointers that I can give, cliché as they sound, but ultimately those are the formulae to be healthy.

Advance Care Plan, Communication that Matters

"Man is the child of customs, not the child of his ancestors."
- Ibn Khaldun

Medicine and healthcare come with a spirit of promoting well-being and reducing sufferings. With this spirit, huge medical advancements have taken place over the past century.

Life expectancy increases and societal expectation for a cure with medical therapy heightens. It used to be, a lot of mortality stems from acute illnesses BUT the demography of illnesses has now change. This can be observed in the baby-boomers' generation with long life expectancy.

This change has brought about a new notion. We can see from many books written, for instance, *The Ageing Societies*, which proposed that the aged community can still be productive and contribute to the economy through having young generations learning from their wisdom. There is also a change and increase in retirement age signalling a change in trend with older people continuing to contribute and be productive for a longer term.

While this change is positive, the incidence and prevalence of chronic organ diseases also increase. It is in fact, common to see hospitalised elderlies with chronic organ dysfunctions. They can be frail., their independence is threatened over time and an increase in the community care is required. The quality of life deteriorates and many develop dementia and eventually terminal dementia. The need for institutionalised care increases due to demand for specialised and comprehensive care for the elderlies. We can debate whether this model of care that results in increased longevity, high allocation of health resources for chronic diseases is the right one or not. The fact remains though, that this is the reality in the healthcare system in most developed countries nowadays.

The question then is how far should we go when we treat our elderly patients? How do we make the best decision in the situation where patients can no longer express their wishes? When there is no advance directive or Enduring

Power of Attorney (EPOA) to assist with decisions about longitudinal care and an increase in the level of care and placement, how do we make the best possible decision for patients? In a situation of tense family disputes, how do we avoid compromise in patients' care?

This leads me to share with you my clinical story.

It is about Mrs Harmony (non-de-plume). Mrs Harmony was a 75-year-old, retired nurse, who lived alone and was reasonably independent with her function at home. She could shower and dress all by herself. She received meals-on-wheels and qualified for assistance with shopping and groceries. She took all her medications that were blister-packed and did not require medications supervision. She had supportive family members but they lived quite far.

As a retired nurse, she knew fully well about the medical and hospital environment. This was the place that she spent decades of her life at. Mrs Harmony did not seem all that worried about the admission to hospital this time.

She was admitted to Christchurch Hospital due to exacerbation of her heart failure. Her legs have become more swollen bilaterally, her lungs were wet with fluid giving bilateral crepitations. Her chest X-ray confirmed the case and her Frusemide dose was increased.

Her breathing kept improving on each day and from the list of patients that I had, she was the least I was worried about.

It was a Thursday morning, the day started as usual with morning handover. Being in the winter season with limited numbers of houseman doctors, I started the ward round with two trainee interns attached to the team.

We went to review several patients and eventually reached to see Mrs Harmony. As we flicked through her file, one of the nurses rushed to me and said, *"Ahmad, Mrs Harmony collapsed after few lapses of walking."* It is not uncommon for an elderly patient to have postural hypotension (a drop in blood pressure upon a transition of posture). I rushed to see her, got the nurses to lie her flat with leg elevation to increase venous return.

Something was not quite right with her. Her BP kept going down. I initiated resuscitation - ABCD, ECG, IV line and IV Fluids. Her BP was not fluid responsive. Her ECG showed sinus tachycardia but with no ischaemic changes. She started to become drowsier. I noted that there was no ceiling of care discussed before and with her having several comorbidities, the outcome of resuscitation would not be pretty.

I called her family who felt that she might not want resuscitation but there was no designated EPOA and there was no advance directive in place. I continued coordinating the acute situation but there was no sign of winning. This to me, was most likely to be a pulmonary embolism with obstructive shock. I called my consultant and discussed whether we should do empiric thrombolysis since a CT scan to confirm this would be impossible in this acute situation.

We ended up giving clexane (blood-thinners) only and in the midst of an emergency situation, I asked Mrs Harmony, *"What do you want us to do should you go unconscious?"*. She stared into my eyes and said, *"Please do not resuscitate me and please let me go."* We wheeled her into a side room, changed our approach to supportive care and she passed away 15 minutes later. During her moment of subconsciousness, I phoned her family, put the phone to her ears and let the remaining moment passed with her listening to the voice of her daughter.

It was a humbling, profound and very emotional moment for all including myself, the nurses and trainee interns involved. We were still reasonably fortunate to be able to honour the wish of Mrs Harmony, albeit in a very difficult situation.

The situation is only one of the millions of examples where resuscitation and end-of-life care decision ended up being made during peri-arrest period. When life-threatening situation emerges, the discussion that should have needed deep contemplation has to happen within few minutes, and this is not right.

The question is, how can we do this better? How can we improve our end-of-life model, acknowledging patients' wishes? How do we ensure that the culture and belief of patients are incorporated when caring for them at their end of life?

In New Zealand and other developed countries, a new concept called Advance Care Plan (ACP) has been introduced. Advance Care Plan is a concept where doctors and healthcare workers encourage and empower patients and community members to engage in profound discussion about their lives. The discussion involves getting patients to think about how they would want to be cared for, the cultural and belief influences, the status of resuscitation, the extent of treatment, their wish for organ donation, the holder of Enduring Power of Attorney (EPOA) and so on.

This concept becomes popular. The reason is that, it gives an honour and recognition to patients' wishes for appropriate treatment. Having an ACP provides clinicians and people who look after the patients, the ability to understand their wishes when they can no longer speak for themselves. ACP also becomes very important when there is a conflict in the family, making the eventual decision hard for the clinicians and unfair for the patients being looked after.

ACP is a process rather than only a document. It gets our community members to think about these crucial questions that in a normal situation would not be approached or thought about by some.

For instance, by knowing in advance that Mrs Harmony had indicated that she would not want resuscitation or debility, the medical approach could be personalised appropriately to clinical context and her wishes. The family could be informed to prepare when something untoward happens, the process of end of life care could be initiated sooner and inappropriate resuscitation could be avoided. It also means when she became unwell and her illness protracted, an arrangement could be made for transfer to the place that she wanted so that she could spend the last moment of her life with her loved ones.

This is the beauty of ACP. It encompasses a holistic area of care and ensures that patients are treated as people with individualised wishes and dignity.

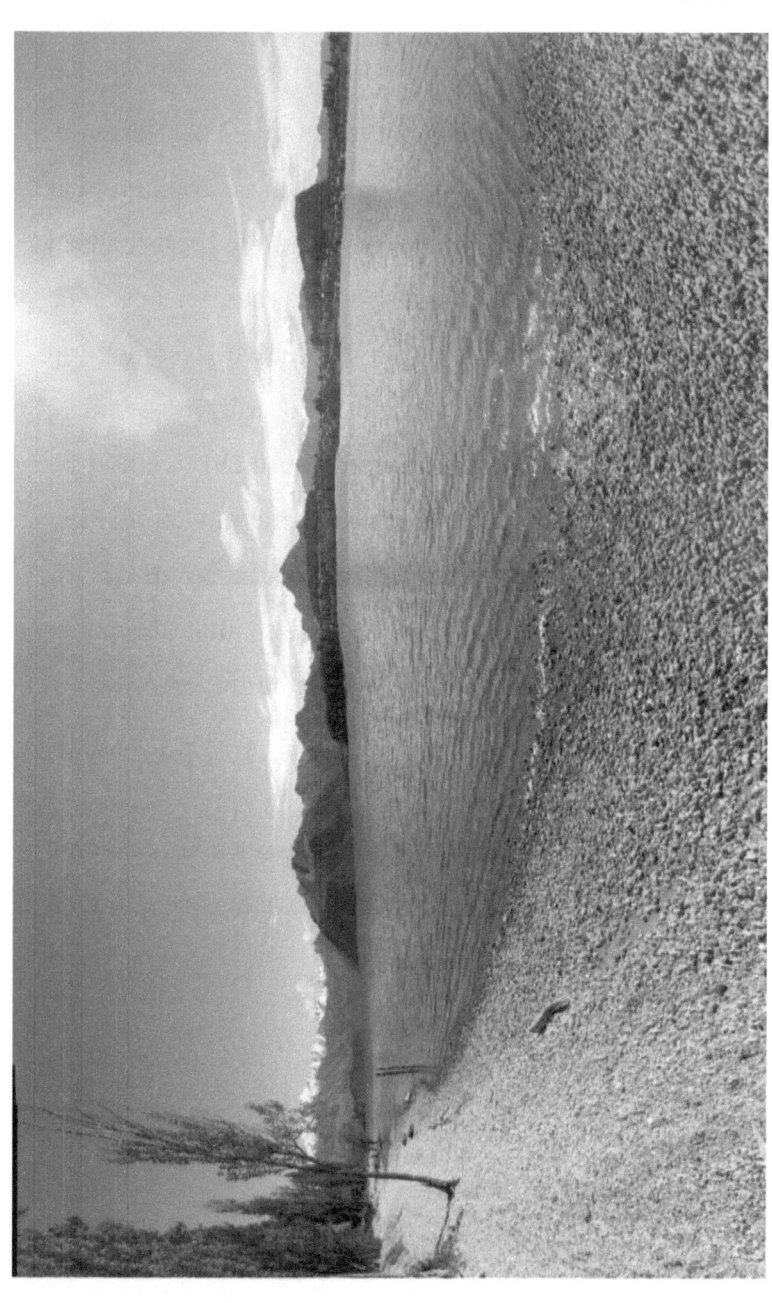

Wanaka, NZ

Cognitive Bias and Clinical Decision Making.

"I am not a product of my circumstances. I am a product of my decisions."– Stephen Covey

The human mind is amazing, for the structure that is complex and for the function which is even more so. From primitive functions to support life, the association of different perceptual stimuli for building of a concept/impression, to the world of psychology unravelling the methodology of thoughts - the spectrum of central neurological functions demands deep contemplation.

I had attended several talks and encountered reading materials on decision-making. They were very interesting and reflected the mechanisms by which decisions were made.

As clinical practitioners, we make a lot of decisions for our patients. Some decisions work best for our patients and some don't. As we experience more, the quality of our decision-making improves, so does the efficiency in making good decisions. What has changed? If we think that the way our brain works could not have changed much except for the formation of long-term potentiation, what could explain this change?

Interestingly, our human mind has two ways by which it derives a judgment/conclusion. Let us call them system A and system B. System A is an effortless, automatic system that creates impression and intuition based on external and internal stimuli. It requires limited effort and creates impression even without us consciously realising it. This is in fact very good because it makes our human mind very efficient in deriving judgment. For instance, when we see a man driving a luxurious car, we would think that he must be a rich man.

System B works by using attention to perform effortful mental activities. It is a very important system, checking the appropriateness of judgment by system A. System B involves deliberation, analysis of available data, proving and disproving hypotheses before a conclusion is reached. It involves laborious effort with eventually less biased conclusion. While this system of thinking is great, it is less efficient and could make clinical decision-making or any decision in life too time-consuming.

Therefore, in most of our decision-making, we employ system A. In the clinical setting, clinicians develop what is called as pattern recognition. This is actually system A, developed over years of clinical experiences. When we see a patient with fever and non-blanching rash, what springs to mind is meningococcal disease. If we see a patient with fever, rash, joint pain and travel history to tropical countries, then dengue or chikungunya would be top of the list.

While system A is great, it is prone to all sorts of biases. A common example is a patient with psychiatric history who presented with shortness of breath. The mind could easily associate this symptom to anxiety given the background history although the organic cause like pneumonia could still likely be the case.

Part of the diagnostic error also comes from this system due to the failure of appropriate diagnostic reasoning. Seeing too many patients with, say, heart failure makes us more likely to think that the next patient with shortness of breath also has heart failure.

The problem is that the biases and an inappropriate conclusion by system A are more noticeable when we listen to others because we are using system B to scrutinise their decisions. Given this is the case, there is a need for awareness about which system is used and for what kind of decision.

A high impact, hard decision will need system B. System A needs to be kept in check when a high impact clinical decision is made.

The Best of Contribution, Filling Life with an Everlasting sense of Giving.

"We make a living by what we get. We make a life by what we give." — Winston S. Churchill

I read a book recently by John Maxwell entitled *Intentional Living*. It was a riveting read, outlining a shift in the way we think about our life. Life is in fact a story. The great thing about it is we can design the story we want and the story that we want to leave for the people that follow after us.

What is great then is the great story that we create by directing ourselves to a particular cause will become a LEGACY for the society. There are many reasons for why we do things. Some people do things for monetary gain. Some would do them for status and position, others would do for love, network and connection. Some would say, the things they do would give them the sense of personal gratification.

Whatever we do, eventually, what gives personal happiness and gratification relates to what we give to others whether it is to the family, friends, community or society. The degree of happiness, gratification and the wealth, interestingly, relates to our degree of contribution to others rather than merely personal gain.

Due to that, the practice of contributing exists and is embedded in every community and society in this world. Contribution is the source for showing kindness, care, love and empathy.

Nowadays, there are a myriad of things being contributed to try to meet the needs of specific groups. If we take the example of UNICEF, the organisation has been providing a range of help to the children in need around the world. From shelters and blankets to education, there are huge areas offered by the organisation to plant the seed of life and hopefully, a better future for the kids in turmoil parts of the world.

Our societies in the developed and developing world have moved further ahead. The increase in life expectancy means that people live longer but suffer from chronic diseases. People, whether they are young adults or older develop end-stage organ problems. With these, the knowledge of organ and tissue transplantation also evolve to allow for human to human transplant.

There are different types of organs and tissues that can be donated and transplanted nowadays. They include heart, heart valves, lungs, kidneys, pancreas, intestines and liver. There are also tissues for transplantation such as cornea and the skin.

The success rate of organ transplantations has also improved. For instance, with the heart, the 5-year organ survival is reaching above 70 percent and it is higher with kidney transplant.

Thinking about how the area of transplantation has evolved and provided people with more hope, I felt strongly called to advocate for people to be organ donors.

I still remember, one day, while I was driving to work, I listened to a story being told on the radio. A lady who suffered from a congenital heart disease since her childhood came to the stage of requiring a heart transplant. She was a young lady full of dreams. Her aspirations to be successful, to get married and to taste the beauty of life were hindered by the limitation of her health. Her fate miraculously changed when to her surprise, a cadaveric donor heart became available and was offered to her. It was from a deceased man who was about the age of her father and who in his life had kindly agreed and signed up for organ donation. She eventually got the transplanted organ.

On her wedding day, as she walked down the aisle, she said *"I really feel thankful, for this heart that feels like the heart of my father."* How beautiful kindness and contribution can be, changing others' lives completely and giving a chance to people like in her situation to enjoy and experience life.

I thought I should carve it in this book, how important and in need we are for organ donation and transplant. Previously, contribution can be made through money, services and help. All these transform people's lives. Nowadays, this transformation can go further to an unimaginable life-changing situation for some people. It is one of the best ways we can serve humanity. Donating organs at the verge of life and death would allow for more people in need to benefit from them. If there is one last thing that we can contribute, why shouldn't it be organ donation?

Organ donor registration varies from country to country, the process can be referred to each country's official organ donation website. If we have a chance to create our great story of life as a legacy, why not ending the chapter of the book by a deed of organ donation.

Updates in the Field of Cancer.

"Challenges are what make life interesting and overcoming them is what makes life meaningful." – Joshua J. Marine

Cancer can be one of the most feared diagnosis that people could have. The reason being, it is notorious for changing the life expectancy and importantly, it dramatically changes the way people live, their psychology, their hope and their expectations.

The troubling thing about cancer is, for most types of advanced cancers, there is no eventual cure.

I spent one weekend attending the Science of Oncology Program organised by the Medical Oncology Group of Australia (MOGA). International and Australian leading experts in the field of oncological sciences were gathered to provide some insights for the trainees in terms of where we are heading in our understanding about cancer.

Why is this important?

As Sun Tzu mentioned:

If you know the enemy and know yourself, you need not fear the result of a hundred battles. If you know yourself but not the enemy, for every victory gained you will also suffer a defeat. If you know neither the enemy nor yourself, you will succumb in every battle.

To understand cancer is to go back to basic cellular biology. Interestingly, the cellular biology is far more complicated than organ functions and physiology. There are millions of cellular pathways, 3 billion human genomic codes and there are mutations to these codes.

Some of the updates that will affect our understanding about cancer for the decades to come:

1. The understanding of the genome and the ability to assess them have been more and more refined such that there are so many new techniques for genetic analyses. These have allowed for identification of what's called driver mutations, passenger mutations, mutational frequency and genetic instability of cancer cells.

2. Cancer mass, in fact, acts like a new organ. It has its own progenitor stem cells and more differentiated cells. This is what's called cancer cell heterogeneity. The cancer cells also have plasticity i.e. the ability to change the surface proteins and causing avoidance/ resistance to treatment.

3. The field of targeted therapies has expanded and looked into the ideas of cell survival and

how to alter them. These include DNA damage and repair, inducing pro-apoptosis, targeting driver mutations rather than passenger mutations, etc.

4. There is now a big appreciation to the phylogenetics of cancer, i.e. why cancer develops progression or becomes resistant to treatment after some time and why recurring cancer could have a different genetic profile? Interestingly, some cancers have very high mutational frequency, hence starting from one clonal cell, as it forms secondary and tertiary metastases, the genetic mutation could be very different from the first clonal cells. For that reason, solid organ biopsy for characterisation of cancer per se would not be accurate in predicting the response to treatment. To increase the detection of responsible driver mutations, sampling circulating DNA, what's

also called liquid biopsy would be more and more commonly done in the near future.

5. The classification of cancers is also now transforming. It was found that the anatomical classification of cancers per se could be misleading. For instance, in gynaecology cancers, different types of ovarian cancers might be completely unrelated. Some, in fact, was due to clonal cell metastases from the gastrointestinal tract. What was found, molecular and genetic classification of cells would be far more accurate in predicting the nature and behaviour of cancers. For instance, triple negative breast cancer and serous ovarian cancer are very closely associated genetically compared to those cancers within their anatomical groups.

Essentially, as research has been discovering further, there are more questions raised than answered. Could it be then the treatment of cancers need to be like HIV treatment, with multi-modality targeted therapies to block several pathways instantaneously and reducing the risk of resistance to treatment?

The approach to fighting cancers has evolved further. While traditionally cancers were associated with multiple genetic mutations that happen in cells, oncologists and oncology clinician-scientists have appreciated what's called the **hallmarks of cancer**.

What's additionally ground-breaking, the realisation that the evolution of cancer cells could happen without changes in DNA mutations. Take, for instance, acute myeloid leukaemia, the recurrent refractory leukemic cells following treatment could occur without new mutational change in the DNA. The question is, how did that happen? This is where the new area called epigenetics comes in. The resistance of cancer cells can be due to epigenetic changes, leading to switching on of different codes of the DNA without changing the DNA sequence in the cell itself.

Given this is the case, the area of targeted therapy opens to more parallel pathways of treatment, targeting the genes and also targeting the epigenetic proteins.

One thing for sure, it goes into never-ending cycles when scrutinising the cellular pathways, the epigenetics, the cancer metabolism and targeting the DNA process. The knowledge for discovery to invent a novel treatment is wide as the ocean.

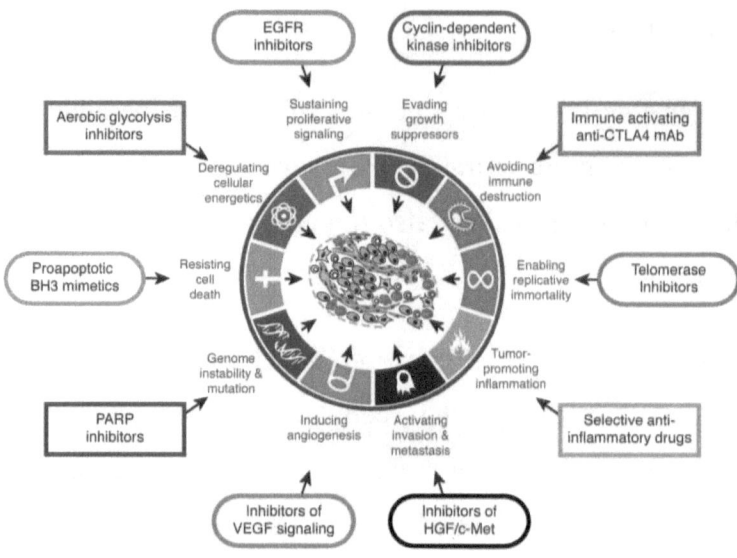

Figure 1: Hallmarks of Cancer.

Revisiting the World of Mental Health.

"Your task is not to seek for love, but merely to seek and find all the barriers within yourself that you have built against it." - Rumi

I had the opportunity to revisit the world of psychiatry and psychology.

A few years ago, when I was in medical school, psychiatry was one of the rotations I loved. The reason being, psychiatry deals with the part of the human self that goes beyond usual scientific reasoning. Fifty to sixty years ago, patients with psychiatric illnesses were presumed to be "possessed". The curiosity into what actually causes these problems and their different manifestations in different cultures (cultural-bound syndromes) had persuaded me to attend the psychiatric conference *"The Wind of Change"*, in late 2012.

During that time, a retired American psychiatrist shared with me at lunch time that functional MRIs were done a lot in research setting to study the psychiatric conundrums. A lot of research in psychology, personality and neurobiology help us nowadays to get some ideas about different groups of psychiatric illnesses including mood disorders, psychotic disorders, anxiety disorders and personality disorders.

From DSM-I to DSM-V, the latter one was published in late 2012, the disorders were described based on their characters but not explaining precisely their pathobiology. In other words, we haven't got the full explanation as to the WHY.

I reviewed many patients in the past when I did my psychiatry rotation and tried to find the common themes among these patients. The life story of people afflicted with mental illness could be saddening.

While yes, the neurotransmitter changes in the brain have roles to play, as well as certain brain areas like frontal lobe and limbic system, it cannot be denied that the environmental, social, upbringings and family factors play huge influence.

For instance, I saw a case of a teenager who grew up in a family with a strong suicidal history who ended up attempting suicide too. Another case was of a person who was born and grew up in a family of prisoners, he ended up in prison too.

Different types of abuse during childhood years have tremendous influence and predisposed the affected individuals to the development of psychiatric illnesses. The other side of the coin as I see it is, the abuses that occurred since the childhood age could impair the ability of those affected to deal with different colours and contrast in life. This is because their worldview and perceptions were already coloured by the negative tragedy at a very young age.

It could well be that the black tragedy as mentioned moulded the brain and psychology of those affected, leading to formation of mature neural wirings in the brain that perpetuated certain mood and behaviours, hence forming the disorders. It is not uncommon that when you ask and try to understand the reasoning of why a person falls into Major Depressive Episode, you might not get the answer. The pain and sufferings were so deep that the reasons were not able to surface to help you understand. The person was locked into their automated mood which was self-perpetuating. This is very different from mere sadness and frustration felt on day to day basis.

I had a patient who tried to hang herself in the hospital bedroom and could only keep repeating *"I am frustrated with my life"* when asked about the reason.

I was listening to Simon Sinek, business and management theorist, on Law of Diffusion of Innovation. This law was originally proposed by

Professor Everett Rogers in 1962. The law stated that any innovation started with an innovator, which then diffused into early adopters, then the early majority, late majority and lastly laggards. The important question for a successful innovator is always about *"Why do you want to do something?"*. The "why" is what created the belief and conviction, from "why" comes "how" to achieve. From there comes "what", which is the product and innovation eventually being developed.

The question of "why" is a life-changing question. The stronger the "why", the more is the "what" that we will become. Perhaps, the environment that one lives in, the education and upbringing that does not necessarily put an emphasis on finding the "why", easily predisposes us to no clear direction. As a result, our organic development and inculcation of values can be impaired. The sense of no purpose because of no "why" can make life very vulnerable and easily taken over and shaped by specific social and environmental exposure.

Perhaps, the innovation in the treatment of certain psychiatric illnesses can be a reconnection to the new WHY to give a new sense of purpose that patients can embody in defining their identity.

Structure and Approach to Care for Patients – A Guide for Interns.

"Courage is the first of human qualities because it is the quality which guarantees all others." - Winston Churchill

Managing patients with medical illnesses is a challenging job. It gets more challenging especially when the illnesses are severe. It is also challenging because a lot of our patients nowadays, presented with multiple co-morbidities which then cause competing priorities. What adds to that situation is, doctoring combines the evidence-based sciences and the art of personalised care for our patients.

Therefore, there should be an approach to ensure safe and good care when patients are in our hands. This is also especially true for the young doctors. Having just graduated from medical school, some might be in shock and uncertain about what to do and how to handle patients better. In some hospitals, the gap and the hierarchal relationship between the junior and senior doctors would mean, it is not as easy to consult or to confess our mistakes.

For that matter, I wrote a simplified guideline to assist the young doctors especially during their first couple of years as house officers or interns.

The first key to managing any patient is to ask yourself, is the patient well or unwell? By that, I mean is the patient rapidly deteriorating or in a life-threatening situation?

By answering this, then you will come to the very question, how far would I/my team go into treating and trying to save the life of this person? This is what we call as the ceiling of care.

How do you determine the ceiling of care? Firstly, if a patient has a recorded advanced directive of do not resuscitate or not for ICU order, then it makes it much clearer.

If none of these is yet available or discussed, then the analysis is on patient's usual functional status, number and extent of co-morbidities, the severity of current illness and the thought of whether the illness is reversible or not. Age also plays a part but is certainly not the only factor.

This will guide the medical decision about the ceiling of care and can be discussed with the ICU and the consultant caring for the patient.

Knowing the ceiling of care, then approach to management of patients can be divided into several categories:

1. Stabilisation - DRS ABCD. This is about calling for the medical emergency team and active cardio/respiratory resuscitation of the patient.

2. Management of symptoms. Once the patient is stabilised, it is important to manage the symptoms that lead to sufferings of the patient. This could be the pain, shortness of breath, nausea and vomiting, temperature and sweats, dizziness or vertigo, etc.

3. Treatments of the underlying conditions. Treatments of the underlying conditions involve formulating hypotheses and clinical reasoning based on clinical history, examination and investigation results. It also involves thinking about the worst-case scenario in an ambiguous situation and ensuring treatment will cover for that. Now, the hypotheses are what we call provisional/ differential diagnoses. If a treatment does not lead to intended improvement, the provisional diagnosis may need to be revisited again and further investigations are carried out to test other hypotheses.

4. Management/prevention of direct or indirect complications. With diseases, complications can develop. For instance, pneumonia can lead to parapneumonic effusion or Acute Respiratory Distress Syndrome (ARDS).

Ischaemic stroke can lead to haemorrhagic transformation. Immobility from paraplegia can lead to the development of deep vein thrombosis. Anticipating the possibility of all these can lead to further action to reduce the risk. For instance, the use of subcutaneous Enoxaparin to prevent deep vein thrombosis (clot in the leg).

5. Assessment of functional status, social situation and mood. While all of the above are important, this part is really the human and defining part that dictates whether a patient can go home or not. Decrease in functional status due to illness can make the ability to live independently difficult. It affects the safety and lead to an unsuccessful discharge planning. Therefore, this part needs good attention and routinely, will need the involvement of multidisciplinary team

including the social worker, physiotherapist and occupational therapist. Remember, hospital is a controlled environment, the situation is completely different at home. Therefore, ensuring good support and help in place before discharging patients would help for successful care for patients.

All the best!

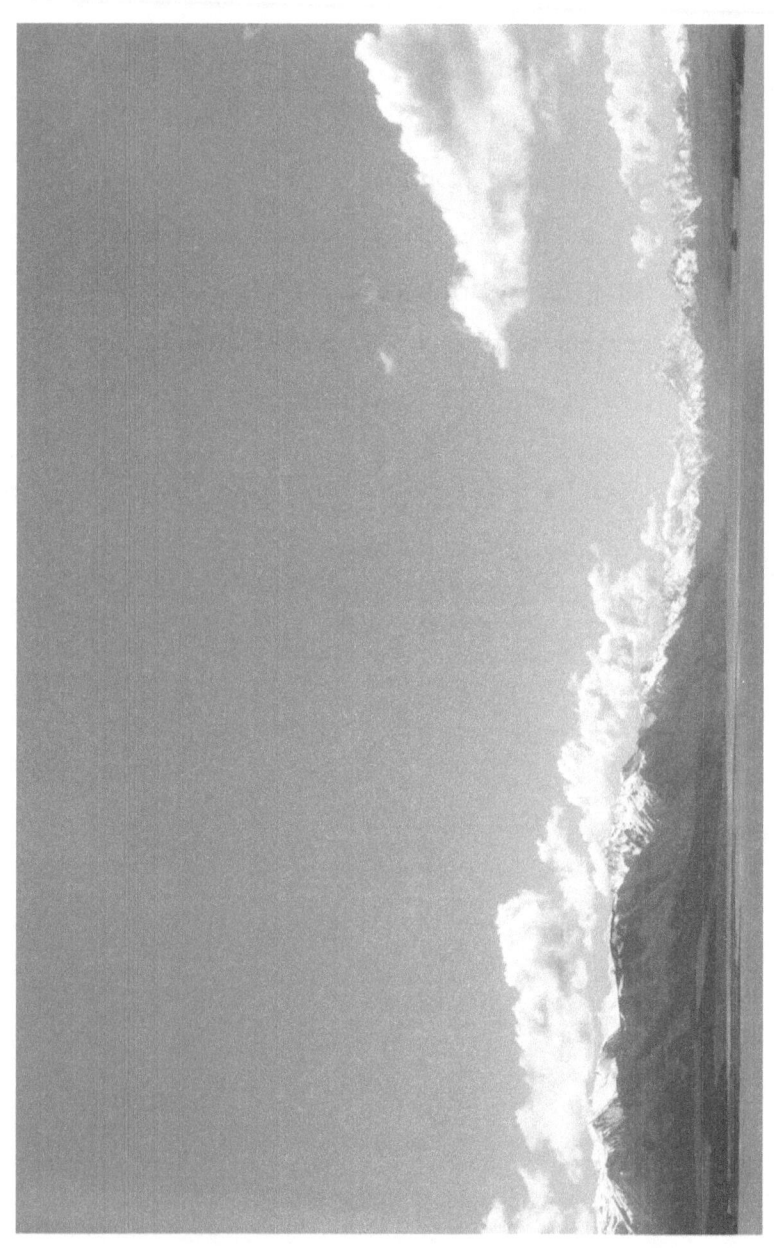

Lake Pukaki, New Zealand

Biography

I was born in Klang, in the state of Selangor, Malaysia. Growing up in a non-medical family, my passion in medicine began after my high school years. I proceeded with Health Science Year in 2007, then my medical degree, MB ChB in Dunedin School of Medicine, University of Otago, NZ from 2008 till 2012.

I did my trainee internship in Dunedin for a year prior to graduation. Following that, I worked two years as a House Officer at Christchurch Hospital, NZ. During my second year of housemanship, I joined the Royal Australasian College of Physician, RACP as a physician trainee.

I sat my physician exam in 2017 and passed both the written and clinical exams, then started my advanced training program since.

I've spent my working years so far enriching my experience in clinical medicine. I've done locum jobs in the rural area, secondary hospital and primary care practice on top of my routine job at tertiary centre. The reason was for me to get a good grasp of clinical experience working in different settings and level of care. Such experience has helped me to evaluate the doctor-patient relationship well in different settings.

Throughout the years of doctoring, part of my interest has been to explore the values that make a doctor a great health professional. My first audit was done in 2013 about 'What makes a good doctor?' which demonstrated discrepancy between doctors and nurses' perspectives on this matter.

My interest has also been in communication skills and resilience in medicine. I attended few courses on these including Level 2 Advance Care Planning(ACP).

I am a believer that medicine needs to be communicated through values. For that reason, I started a sole proprietorship and started selling my stethoscope brand 'Listen2Heart' on Amazon in 2016-2017. Having tested the market, I am now eager to spread the message of communicating medicine through values. This book, *Two Sides of the World: Doctors and Patients* is one of the avenues to achieving that.

Bibliography

Topic 1

Hill, Napoleon, 2004: *Think and Grow Rich*, USA : The Random House Publishing Group.

Robbins, Anthony, 1992: *Awaken the Giant Within*, USA: Free Press.

Success Magazine ; www.success.com.

Rohn, Jim,: *My Philosophy for Successful Living*, 2012, USA: No Dream too Big LLC.

Ma, Jack: *How to be Successful in you 20,30,40s and beyond*: https://www.cnbc.com/2018/01/30/jack-ma-dont-fear-making-mistakes-in-your-20s-and-30s.html

Maxwell, John, 2015: *Intentional Living, Choosing a Life that Matters*, USA : Center Street.

TED Talks; https://www.ted.com/talks.

Clason, George Samuel, 2002 : *The Richest Man in Babylon*, USA : Berkeley.

Roberts RC. The blessings of gratitude: a conceptual analysis. In: Emmons RA, McCullough ME, eds. The

Psychology of Gratitude. New York: Oxford University Press; 2004:58–78. 3.

Fredrickson BL. Gratitude, like other positive emotions, broadens and builds. In: Emmons RA, McCullough ME, (eds). The Psychology of Gratitude. New York: Oxford University Press; 2004:145–166.

Topic 2

Goodwin, C. (2016). Person-Centered Care: A Definition and Essential Elements. *Journal of the American Geriatrics Society*, *64*(1), 15–18. https://doi.org/10.1111/jgs.13866

Ha, J. F., & Longnecker, N. (2010). Doctor-patient communication: a review. *The Ochsner Journal*, *10*(1), 38–43. https://doi.org/10.1043/toj-09-0040.1

Kirkcaldy, B. D., Shephard, R. J., & Siefen, R. G. (2010). *The making of a good doctor. The Making of a Good Doctor*. Retrieved from https://www.scopus.com/inward/record.uri?eid=2-

s2.0-84895231763&partnerID=40&md5=289cf96852aedf472a605eb09122cbd2

Tsou, A. Y., Creutzfeldt, C. J., & Gordon, J. M. (2013). The good doctor: Professionalism in the 21st century. *Handbook of Clinical Neurology, 118*, 119–132. https://doi.org/10.1016/B978-0-444-53501-6.00009-3

Topic 3

Robinson, Ken, 2009 : *The Element: How Finding Your Passion Changes Everything*, USA : Penguin.

Topic 4

Pilcher JJ, Huffcutt AI. Effects of sleep deprivation on performance: a meta-analysis. Sleep 1996;19:318–26.

Agency for Healthcare Research and Quality. The effect of health care working conditions on patient safety. Evidence Report/Technology Assessment No. 74.

Rockville (MD): AHRQ; 2003. Available at: http://www.ncbi.nlm.nih.gov/books/NBK36875/.

Paul Kalanithi; When Breath Becomes Air.

Topic 5

Lown, Bernard, 1999: *The Lost Art of Healing, Practicing Compassion in Medicine*, USA: The Random House of Publishing Group.

Diener E, Seligman ME. Beyond money. Toward an economy of well-being. *Psychological Science in the Public Interest* 2004;5(1):1–31.

Diener E. Assessing well-being: the collected works of Ed Diener. New York: Springer; 2009.

Diener E, Scollon CN, Lucas RE. The evolving concept of subjective well-being: the multifaceted nature of happiness. In: E Diener (ed.) *Assessing well-being: the collected works of Ed Diener*. New York: Springer; 2009:67–100.

Frey BS, Stutzer A. Happiness and economics. Princeton, N.J.: Princeton University Press; 2002.

Diener E, Lucas R, Schimmack U, and Helliwell J. Well-Being for public policy. New York: Oxford University Press; 2009.

Topic 6

Arem, H., Moore, S. C., Patel, A., Hartge, P., de Gonzalez, A. B., Visvanathan, K., ... Matthews, C. E. (2015). Leisure Time Physical Activity and Mortality: A Detailed Pooled Analysis of the Dose-Response Relationship. *JAMA Internal Medicine*, *175*(6), 959–967. https://doi.org/10.1001/jamainternmed.2015.0533

Beaglehole, R., & Bonita, R. (2009). Alcohol: a global health priority. *The Lancet*, *373*(9682), 2173–2174. https://doi.org/10.1016/S0140-6736(09)61168-5

Berkman, N. D., Sheridan, S. L., Donahue, K. E., Halpern, D. J., & Crotty, K. (2011). Low health literacy and health outcomes: An updated systematic review. *Annals of Internal Medicine*. https://doi.org/10.7326/0003-4819-155-2-201107190-00005

Chodzko-Zajko, W. J., Proctor, D. N., Fiatarone Singh,

M. A., Minson, C. T., Nigg, C. R., Salem, G. J., & Skinner, J. S. (2009). Exercise and physical activity for older adults. *Medicine and Science in Sports and Exercise.* https://doi.org/10.1249/MSS.0b013e3181a0c95c

Fagerström, K. (2002). The epidemiology of smoking: health consequences and benefits of cessation. *Drugs, 62 Suppl 2,* 1–9. https://doi.org/10.2165/00003495-200262002-00001

Kalager, M., Zelen, M., Langmark, F., & Adami, H.-O. (2010). Effect of Screening Mammography on Breast-Cancer Mortality in Norway. *New England Journal of Medicine, 363*(13), 1203–1210. https://doi.org/10.1056/NEJMoa1000727

Kickbusch, I., Pelikan, J., Apfel, F., & Tsouros, a. (2013). Health literacy: the solid facts. *Copenhagen: WHO Regional Office for ...,* 7–8. https://doi.org/10.1016/j.socscimed.2008.09.050

Kirk-Sanchez, N. J., & McGough, E. L. (2014). Physical exercise and cognitive performance in the elderly: current perspectives. *Clinical Interventions in Aging, 9*, 51–62. https://doi.org/10.2147/CIA.S39506

Kokkinos, P., & Myers, J. (2010). Exercise and physical activity: Clinical outcomes and applications. *Circulation*. https://doi.org/10.1161/CIRCULATIONAHA.110.948349

Mizowaki, Y., Sugawara, S., Yamamoto, K., Sakamoto, Y., Iwagaki, Y., Kawakami, Y., … Tsuduki, T. (2017). Comparison of the Effects of the 1975 Japanese Diet and the Modern Mediterranean Diet on Lipid Metabolism in Mice. *Journal of Oleo Science, 66*(5), 507–519. https://doi.org/10.5650/jos.ess16241

Mulatu, M. S., & Schooler, C. (2002). Causal Connections between Socio-Economic Status and Health: Reciprocal Effects and Mediating Mechanisms. *Journal of Health and Social Behavior, 43*(1), 22. https://doi.org/10.2307/3090243

National Institute on Alcohol Abuse and Alcoholism. (2000). Health risks and benefits of alcohol consumption. *The Journal of the National Institute on Alcohol Abuse and Alcoholism, 24*(1), 5–11.

Osborn, C. Y., Paasche-Orlow, M. K., Bailey, S. C., & Wolf, M. S. (2011). The mechanisms linking health literacy to behavior and health status. *American Journal of Health Behavior, 35*(1), 118–128.

Peluso, M. A. M., & Guerra de Andrade, L. H. S. (2005). Physical activity and mental health: the association between exercise and mood. *Clinics (Sao Paulo, Brazil), 60*(1), 61–70. https://doi.org/10.1590/S1807-59322005000100012

Penedo, F. J., & Dahn, J. R. (2005). Exercise and well-being: A review of mental and physical health benefits associated with physical activity. *Current Opinion in Psychiatry.* https://doi.org/10.1097/00001504-200503000-00013

Pomerleau, J., Pederson, L. L., Ostbye, T., Speechley, M., & Speechley, K. N. (1997). Health behaviours and socio-economic status in Ontario, Canada. *European Journal of Epidemiology,* 13(6), 613–622.

https://doi.org/10.1023/A:1007339720807

Rehm, J., Gmel, G., Sempos, C. T., & Trevisan, M. (2003). Alcohol-related morbidity and mortality. *Alcohol Research & Health: The Journal of the National Institute on Alcohol Abuse & Alcoholism, 27*(1), 39–51. https://doi.org/Retrieved from http://www.ncbi.nlm.nih.gov/pubmed/15301399

Samet, J. M. (1991). Health benefits of smoking cessation. *Clin Chest Med, 12*(4), 669–679. https://doi.org/10.1164/ajrccm/142.5.993

Shaukat, A., Mongin, S. J., Geisser, M. S., Lederle, F. A., Bond, J. H., Mandel, J. S., & Church, T. R. (2013). Long-term mortality after screening for colorectal cancer. *The New England Journal of Medicine, 369*(12), 1106–1114. https://doi.org/10.1056/NEJMoa1300720

Sofi, F., Cesari, F., Abbate, R., Gensini, G. F., & Casini, A. (2008). Adherence to Mediterranean diet and health status: meta-analysis. *BMJ (Clinical Research Ed.)*. https://doi.org/10.1136/bmj.a1344

Sofi, F., Macchi, C., Abbate, R., Gensini, G. F., & Casini,

A. (2013). Mediterranean diet and health. *BioFactors*. https://doi.org/10.1002/biof.1096

T??nnesen, P. (2013). Smoking cessation and COPD. *European Respiratory Review*. https://doi.org/10.1183/09059180.00007212

Taylor, C. B., Sallis, J. F., & Needle, R. (1985). The relation of physical activity and exercise to mental health. *Public Health Reports (Washington, D.C. : 1974)*, *100*(2), 195–202. Retrieved from http://www.ncbi.nlm.nih.gov/pubmed/3920718%5Cnhttp ://www.pubmedcentral.nih.gov/articlerender.fcgi?artid= PMC1424736%5Cnhttp://www.pubmedcentral.nih.gov/a rticlerender.fcgi?artid=1424736&tool=pmcentrez&rende rtype=abstract

Trichopoulou, A., Martínez-González, M. A., Tong, T. Y. N., Forouhi, N. G., Khandelwal, S., Prabhakaran, D., … de Lorgeril, M. (2014). Definitions and potential health benefits of the Mediterranean diet: Views from experts around the world. *BMC Medicine*, *12*(1). https://doi.org/10.1186/1741-7015-12-112

Vlismas, K., Stavrinos, V., & Panagiotakos, D. B. (2009). Socio-economic status, dietary habits and health-related outcomes in various parts of the world: A review. *Central European Journal of Public Health, 17*(2), 55–63.

Warburton, D. E. R., Nicol, C. W., & Bredin, S. S. D. (2006). Health benefits of physical activity: the evidence. *CMAJ : Canadian Medical Association Journal = Journal de l'Association Medicale Canadienne, 174*(6), 801–809. https://doi.org/10.1503/cmaj.051351=

Topic 7

Hooper, Sarah, 2006: *Ageing Societies*, USA: Hodder Arnold Publication.

Advance Care Planning; http://www.advancecareplanning.org.nz/ .

Topic 8

Kahneman, Daniel, 2011: *Thinking, Fast and Slow*, USA : FSG.

Banning, M. (2008). A review of clinical decision making: Models and current research. *Journal of Clinical Nursing, 17*(2), 187–195. https://doi.org/10.1111/j.1365-2702.2006.01791.x

Croskerry, P. (2002). Achieving quality in clinical decision making: cognitive strategies and detection of bias. *Acad Emerg Med, 9*(11), 1184–1204. https://doi.org/10.1111/j.1553-2712.2002.tb01574.x

Topic 9

Maxwell, John, 2015: *Intentional Living, Choosing a Life that Matters*, USA : Center Street.

Lodhi, S. A., & Meier-Kriesche, H.-U. (2011). Kidney allograft survival: the long and short of it. *Nephrology Dialysis Transplantation, 26*(1), 15–17. Retrieved from http://dx.doi.org/10.1093/ndt/gfq730

Shahbazi, F., Ranjbaran, M., Karami-far, S., Soori, H., & Manesh, H. J. (2015). Graft survival rate of renal transplantation during a period of 10 years in Iran. *Journal of Research in Medical Sciences : The Official Journal of Isfahan University of Medical Sciences*, *20*(11), 1046–1052. https://doi.org/10.4103/1735-1995.172814

Wilhelm, M. J. (2015). Long-term outcome following heart transplantation: current perspective. *Journal of Thoracic Disease*, *7*(3), 549–551. https://doi.org/10.3978/j.issn.2072-1439.2015.01.46

Topic 10

Sun Tzu, 2002: *The Art of War*, USA: Dover Publications.

Hallmarks of Cancer: The Next Generation, Hanahan, Douglas et al. Cell, Volume 144, Issue 5 , 646 – 674.

Gay, L., Baker, A.-M., & Graham, T. A. (2016). Tumour Cell Heterogeneity. *F1000Research*, *5*, F1000 Faculty Rev-238. https://doi.org/10.12688/f1000research.7210.1

Peng, W. (2012). Tumor phylogenetics. *Nature Genetics*, *44*, 368. Retrieved from http://dx.doi.org/10.1038/ng.2240

Pon, J. R., & Marra, M. A. (2015). Driver and Passenger Mutations in Cancer. *Annual Review of Pathology: Mechanisms of Disease*, *10*(1), 25–50. https://doi.org/10.1146/annurev-pathol-012414-040312

Sharma, S., Kelly, T. K., & Jones, P. A. (2010). Epigenetics in cancer. *Carcinogenesis*, *31*(1), 27–36. https://doi.org/10.1093/carcin/bgp220

Topic 11

Sinek, Simon, 2009: Start with Why, How Great Leaders Inspire Everyone to Take Action, USA: Penguin.

LaMorte, Wayne W. , 2016 : *Diffusion of Innovation Theory*, Boston University of Public Health : Accessed in 2016 via URL : http://sphweb.bumc.bu.edu/otlt/MPH-Modules/SB/BehavioralChangeTheories/BehavioralChangeTheories4.html

www.ingramcontent.com/pod-product-compliance
Lightning Source LLC
Chambersburg PA
CBHW020436220526
45464CB00002B/726